TRAUMA INFORMED APPROACH
A SAMHSA MODEL IN CUSTODY

Selma De Jesús-Zayas, Ph.D.
Director, Mental Health
Creative Corrections

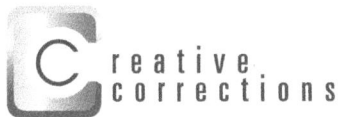

creative
corrections

De Jesús-Zayas, Ph.D., Selma.
   Trauma Informed Approach A SAMHSA Model In Custody.

Printed in the United States of America

Preface

It was not that long ago that women and children who reported sexual abuse were thought to be lying and their trauma related symptoms ignored (Jordan,2004; Trauma Informed Care in Behavioral Services, 2014). However, thanks to the Substance Abuse and Mental Health Services Administration ("SAMHSA"), a series of incisive research projects sponsored by them exposed how widespread and pernicious is this problem. Not only was victimization much more prevalent in society, males were just as likely as females and children to experience victimization.

An additional finding was how institutions geared toward helping victims of trauma inadvertently implemented procedures or methodology that re-traumatized those they were serving. In response to these findings, SAMHSA developed a philosophy and treatment modality they recommend be implemented in all agencies to ensure early detection of trauma victims and prevention of re-traumatization.

Correctional facilities are just as likely as any mental health and medical agencies to receive individuals who are experiencing trauma related symptoms. It is incumbent upon a correctional institution to be cognizant of trauma related symptoms and address them to avoid further re-traumatization. In addition, it would be a sound correctional practice as this intervention would enable staff to maintain an orderly and secure operation that otherwise might have been compromised due to the individual's trauma-related disruptive behavior.

This book serves three purposes: 1) Teach the philosophy and concepts of a Trauma Informed Approach ("TIA") 2) Integrate the TIA approach to a correctional environment 3) Offer a training modality to those who will then train others.

We hope you find this information to be useful and that you are able to successfully train staff as well as implement this philosophy at your institution.

Selma De Jesús-Zayas, Ph.D.
December 1, 2016

TABLE OF CONTENTS

TRAUMA INFORMED APPROACH
A SAMHSA MODEL IN CUSTODY

INTRODUCTION

According to the Substance Abuse and Mental Health Services, (2012) "trauma" is a widespread occurrence that results in a plethora of mental health and physical ailments. It is so widespread that unless addressed these medical and mental health conditions can strain our society by placing extraordinary burdens on families, work settings, and institutions.

In Custody, inmates might display trauma related disruptive behaviors that unless recognized for what they are will continue to perpetuate themselves and most likely lead to interventions that result in re-traumatization. In addition, these behaviors place an additional burden on Custody staff. Custody staff, however, are in a position to identify trauma related behaviors, address them, as well as avoid engaging in discipline measures that might lead to re-traumatizing.

The "Trauma Informed Approach" ("TIA") recognizes "the widespread impact of trauma and understands the (different) potential paths for recovery; recognizes the signs and symptoms of trauma in clients, families, staff, and others involved with the system; and responds by fully integrating knowledge about trauma into policies, procedures, and practices, and seeks to actively resist re-traumatization". (2014, p. 9). It is the purpose of this presentation to integrate the concepts of a TIA philosophy with the needs and mission of a correctional facility while teaching trainers who in turn will train correctional staff the principles of a TIA modality.

PURPOSE

This Training for Trainers ("TT") program is based on the beliefs, principles, and recommendations issued by The Substance Abuse and Mental Health Services Administration ("SAMHSA") regarding Trauma Informed Approach ("TIA"). These principles are found in their Treatment Improvement Protocol, Tip 57. This program is designed to aid Trainers present these concepts to other trainers who will then teach staff how to implement them in a custody environment. It is critical to understand how to apply, and integrate, TIA concepts in a manner that is consistent with the values and principles of a custody setting.

The program is designed to be an INTERACTIVE course. It is important for participants to become involved in order to better learn the concepts and principles being discussed. To achieve this goal, a series of interactive exercises have been developed at the conclusion of each major section of this program. Trainers need to encourage participation in the form of question and answers; small group interactions; role plays; etc. A suggested format is as follows: From 8:00 A.M. – 12:00 pm, half an hour presentation, followed by a twenty minute small group discussion, another twenty minutes with the larger group, and a ten minute break. From 1:00- 4:30 P.M. half hour small group discussions followed by half hour large group discussions. By all means, make it fun! Improvise with the interactive questions and make it an exciting experience. Good luck!

GOALS

1) Ensure compliance with the Substance Abuse and Mental Health Services Administration's mission to teach all agencies the deleterious effects trauma has on the affected individual, those in contact with the individual, agencies, and society in general.

2) Address how a correctional institution can avoid traumatizing inmates and re-traumatizing those who have already been exposed to a traumatic incident.

3) Learn of the impact trauma-related behaviors may have in a custody environment.

4) Review custody-related interventions and their effect on an inmate with a previous history of trauma.

5) Explore ways of recognizing and addressing disruptive trauma- related behaviors in prison.

6) Explore how to enforce an institution's discipline code while being mindful of TIA's principles.

HISTORY

The Substance Abuse and Mental Health Services Administration ("SAMHSA") is an agency within the U.S. Department of Health and Human Services established by Congress in 1992 to ensure that substance use and mental disorder information, services, and research data are easily accessible to the general population. This agency is tasked with leading public health initiatives designed to advance the nation's behavioral health efforts. Its mission is to "reduce the impact of substance abuse and mental illness" throughout the U.S.("about-us," 2016).

Back in the early 1990's women survivors of traumatic events became vocal about how they were being re-traumatized by the medical and law enforcement communities they went to for assistance. They discussed how in the process of trying to obtain help from law enforcement and/or medical community the standard practices employed at the time simply resulted in triggering memories of the abuse and in re-victimization.

For example, during a typical, routine session with the local police these women found the focus of the interview remained on gathering as much information as possible with little regard for them as victims or for their emotional state. Consequently, many women reported feeling as if they were being abused all over again. Many described the interview process being as disturbing as the original traumatic event itself (National Sexual Violence Resource Center, 2012).

Due to the impact of traumatic events on memory, women's recollections of their traumatic incident were often spotty. As law enforcement officers tried to clarify apparent discrepancies, elicit information, or fill in time gaps, victims often felt as if they were being perceived and treated as being dishonest. Women reported that law enforcement officers often did not find their accounts credible. Women would often leave the interviews feeling as if they were the culprits instead of the victims of a traumatic incident (Jordan, 2004).

In health settings, women reported how the focus was primarily on their medical condition, not on how they were trying to come to terms with their trauma. For example, health professionals would ask them to submit to medical procedures that would unwittingly re-enact the traumatic event (e.g., undressing). Once again, these practices resulted in women feeling as if they were being re-victimized.

In 1994, SAMHSA's "Dare to Vision Conference" became the first conference where women who had survived a traumatic incident met to describe their experiences within the medical setting. Many of these women spoke about how traumatizing their experiences with the medical community had been which led SAMHSA to action. Based on the information gathered at this conference, in 1998, SAMHSA funded the "Women, Co-Occurring Disorders and Violence Study" that helped gather information on the development and evaluation of treatment and specialty services available for women with mental and substance abuse disorders who, in addition, had been physically and/or sexually abused.

As women felt more empowered to speak about their abuse and victimization, support groups emerged giving them additional voice and power. These groups have, in turn, assisted in offering researchers and clinicians additional nuances from which to explore, and learn from, as they expanded their knowledge of victimization and abuse.

Researchers also noted how traumatized individuals could be found within any context in addition to a mental health setting. For example, they identified trauma victims in the criminal and justice system, school settings, the military, etc. This meant that every agency needed to properly identify those who had been victimized to prevent their re-victimization. In custody this directive means that all inmate's need to be assessed to determine if s/he was a victim of a traumatic event but also there needs to be a review of commonly employed procedures (i.e., strip searches, seclusion and restraints) that need to be re-examined within the context of preventing "re-victimization."

One of the major findings obtained from these research projects was how the structure and climate of organizations designed to assist victims overcome by trauma played a central role in maximizing, or not, their recovery. They determined that in order to prevent re-traumatization it was essential for the agency as a whole to fine tune it's interventions and culture to ensure it was not, inadvertently, contributing to the re-traumatization of the victims. Therefore, correctional institutions wishing to implement a TIA modality need to review their operations to determine if they are inadvertently traumatizing or re-traumatizing inmates with their policies, attitudes, behaviors, and discipline measures.

RESEARCH

Research on trauma has a long history but it was not until the inclusion of the diagnosis of Post Traumatic Stress Disorder in the third edition of the Diagnostic and Statistical Manual of Mental Disorders (DSM-III, 1980) that the condition began to achieve some scientific recognition. (The DSM is the authoritative guide to mental disorders used by the mental health profession.) As a result of this diagnosis, additional research was conducted and novel research-based interventions generated.

Initially, a key concept of this diagnosis was the presence of a "triggering event" that was so traumatic it was outside the realm of normal human experience. Presently, a diagnosis of "PTSD" does not require "the presence of a traumatic event outside the realm of normal human experience" to be assigned. Instead, the essential feature is "the development of symptoms after exposure to one or more traumatic events."   Some of these salient symptoms include anger, irritability, flashbacks, memory impairment, negative beliefs and expectations, avoidance of images or experiences that could remind the individual of the traumatic event, startled responses, reckless self-destructive behavior, etc. (DSM-5, 2013, 271-280).

SAMHSA'S DEFINITIONS

Prior to reviewing concepts critical to the understanding of TIA these need to be defined.

Trauma – Individual trauma results from an event, series of events, or set of circumstances that are experienced by an individual as physically or emotionally harmful or life threatening and that has lasting adverse effects on his/her functioning and mental, physical, social, emotional, or spiritual well-being.

The DSM 5's definition differs somewhat from SAMHSA as it defines trauma as "when an individual person is exposed to actual or threatened death, serious injury, or sexual violence" (APA, 2013, p. 271).

Trauma Related Symptoms - these are behaviors that have emerged as the individual tries to cope in the best possible way with their traumatic experience. These symptoms might have functioned at some point in time, might have helped the individual cope with his/her traumatic event, but in different contexts, or different stages in life, these coping skills might no longer be effective. Instead, they might be interfering with the individual's ability to form long lasting intimate relationships, maintain emotional stability, and refrain from substance abuse.

Individual's reacting to trauma might be functioning optimally in some areas and not others. In other words, the individual 's problems might be contained to one area like sleeping difficulty, interpersonal relationships, etc., but while limited in scope it does not mean they are not trauma related symptoms. In other words, individual's reacting to trauma might be functioning optimally in some areas and not others. This variability occurs because individuals who have survived a traumatic event vary in their expression of symptoms and the severity of symptoms.

As part of their recovery process, it is important to focus on the individual's coping and adaptive skills so that instead of perceiving their behavior as "pathological" or "ill" we concentrate on their resiliency and strengths. This means that we begin to view their maladaptive behaviors as normal reactions to abnormal situations which in turn help us stress hope in a better future based on their assets rather than weaknesses.

Complex Trauma: According to the National Child Traumatic Stress Network, (2004) complex trauma is defined as: " a dual problem involving both exposure to traumatic events and the impact of this exposure on immediate and long-term outcomes."

Complex trauma usually involves multiple traumatic incidents (sometimes simultaneously, sometimes sequentially). Research points out that individuals with a protracted and repeated history of traumatic events exhibit more serious cases of PTSD and personality disturbances in general (Ehring and Quack, 2010).

Trauma Informed Approach (equally known as "Trauma Informed Care" or "TIC") – "A program, organization, or system that is trauma-informed realizes the widespread impact of trauma and understands potential paths for recovery: recognizes the signs and symptoms of trauma in clients, families, staff, and others involved with the system; and responds by fully integrating knowledge about trauma into policies, procedures, and practices, and seeks to actively resist re-traumatization" (SAMHSA'S Concept of Trauma and Guidance for a Trauma Informed Approach, 2014,p9).

PREVALENCE

The prevalence of trauma differs according to its context. For example, as recently reported by the World Health Organization

("WHO," 2013), an estimated 3.6% of the world's population suffered from post-traumatic stress disorder in the previous year. They also listed the following incidents as the most traumatic events witnessed or lived: violence (21.8%), experiencing interpersonal violence (18.8%), accidents (17.7%), exposure to war (16.2%), trauma to a loved one (12.5%).

In 2011, the National Epidemiologic Survey on Alcohol and Related Conditions (Pietrzak , et al, 2011) published the results of a large-scale survey assessing behavioral health in the U.S. This survey incorporated 27 different types of potentially traumatic events and they found a lifetime prevalence of Post -traumatic stress disorder or partial PTSD (did not meet all of the criteria for PTSD) of 6.4% with rates being higher for women (8.6%) than for men (4.1%). They also found that the most traumatic events in the U.S. were as follows: Indirect experience of 9/11 terrorist attack against the U.S., serious illness or injury to someone close, and unexpected death of someone close.

For those who wonder why it is that those individuals experiencing trauma related symptoms cannot "think" their way out of them or "snap out" of them, the following presentation from Ted Talks helps to explain this phenomena. This presentation is offered by Dr. John L. Rigg, MD, FAAPMR, who is the Medical Director for NeuroRestorative Georgia and serves as the Traumatic Brain Injury Program Director for the Dwight D. Eisenhower Army Medical Center at Fort Gordon, GA.

https://www.youtube.com/watch?v=m9Pg4K1ZKws

Interactive Questions-
Form small discussion groups to answer these questions and then role play as if discussing with someone who has not participated in the training. Afterward, meet as a large group. Each team will select a representative who will answer each one of these questions in front of the larger group.

> 1- *What is SAMHSA and what does it wish to achieve?*
> 2- *How did SAMHSA give a voice to female victims of trauma?*
> 3- *What is a "triggering event?"*
> 4- *What is PTSD and how has this definition changed through the years?*
> 5- *What is Trauma?*
> 6- *What is a "Trauma Related Symptom?*
> 7- *What is Complex Trauma?*

8- *What is a Trauma Informed Approach and how does it differ from Trauma Informed Care?*

9- *Role play a conscientious correctional officer conducting a pat-down compared to a conscientious correctional officer who has training in TIA conducting the pat down (after chow).*

TIA KEY PRINCIPLES AND CUSTODY

Awareness of the presence of trauma or the understanding of trauma-specific interventions is not enough when treating those who are traumatized. Instead, the CONTEXT in which treatment is being delivered is extremely important to ensure an optimal outcome. This means that trauma-specific interventions cannot be relegated to the medical or mental health division of a prison or jail but that every staff member needs to be able to understand these principles and employ them accordingly. It also means the agency needs to demonstrate commitment to these principles and that its culture and procedures reflect this commitment.

According to SAMHSA, the concept of trauma-informed approach is based on the following four assumptions and six principles that in essence constitute its Guiding Principles: Realization, Recognize, Respond, Resist Re-traumatization.

We are going to look at each one, explain how they might be problematic in a custody environment, and then we will explore how they might be implemented in a correctional setting.

A) **Realization-** For an organization to be considered committed to a "Trauma Informed Approach" each member, at all levels, needs to be aware ("realize") what trauma entails and how it can affect not only the individual but others in contact with, or related to, that individual. They need to be aware that this condition affects not only the victim but those who interact and /or are related to the victim. They also need to be aware that victimization is present in many contexts to include prison, jails, and detention centers. This knowledge is important in a custody setting because trauma could be a key aspect of mental (and substance abuse) disorder that if neglected or dismissed might hinder that person's ability to comply with an institution's regulations and/or result in interventions that require external control measures that might re- traumatize the individual.

B) **Recognize-** At a "Trauma Informed Approach" center each member is able to recognize the symptoms of trauma. As each member becomes informed, they are able to recognize these symptoms and make proper referrals. In custody, staff can be taught how to recognize symptoms through supervision, training, internal newsletters, policy statements, guest speakers, etc.

C) **Responds-** By being aware how traumatic events have a wide reaching impact, each member of organizations committed to a "Trauma Informed Approach" must ensure their services are geared toward providing a psychologically and physically safe environment. This safe environment can be achieved by promoting policies geared toward trauma recovery, and ensuring that staff exhibit "universal precaution" whereby one anticipates those being served have experienced a traumatic event and need to be treated in such a way that would minimize re-traumatization.

D) **Resist Re-Traumatization-** Organizations committed to a "Trauma Informed Approach" need to analyze their protocols to ensure they are not employing interventions that might inadvertently re-traumatize an individual. For example, in a school setting the use of corporal punishment might re-traumatize a child who is being victimized at home. In a medical or mental health setting seclusion and restraints might re-traumatize those with a history of neglect and severe punishments. Therefore, it is important to keep in mind that some of the interventions available in a custody environment might trigger memories of previous trauma.

Inmates who have experienced a traumatic event might react in peculiar ways to certain triggers. Custody staff need to be mindful of these triggers and point these out to the inmate. If staff feel this is not their role, (for example, the refrigeration foreman) they can at least share this information with that inmate's treatment team so they may address it with the inmate. By taking this course of action staff would be intervening in a manner that recognizes the presence of trauma as well as trying to prevent re-traumatization.

A tenet of Trauma Informed Approach is to not ignore patients' symptoms and demands when they "act out" in response to triggered trauma.

In Custody, strict regulations are designed so inmates (and staff) are cognizant of what type of authorized behaviors they may display. (BOP, 2016). These behavioral regulations are implemented with the primary goal of operating a safe and secure institution. Therefore, behaviors that breach these guidelines will most likely not be ignored but instead acknowledged and possibly disciplined. However, custody based interventions could run the high risk of re-traumatizing inmates.

In society, we are able to respond to a person's needs and vulnerabilities with a wider range of interventions than those available in custody. Once an individual enters a correctional facility the range of interventions is restrained by rules and policies that focus primarily on maintaining the institution's integrity, its security. This means that individual needs are secondary to those of the institution. However, if we are working with an inmate with a history of trauma, and we observe a reaction that requires disciplining but that might be trauma-related, an important step would be to consider that person's behavior within the context of the institution as well as the traumatic event. It is important to consider both aspects, the safety of the institution as well as the original traumatic incident, when developing an intervention. Once the inmate's behavior is understood from this perspective decisions can be made that not only address the institution's requirements but the traumatic incident as well. Being cognizant of the institution's demands and the traumatic event will provoke staff to seek novel ways of handling the trauma-related disruptive behavior.

The Trauma Informed Approach warns that when trying to control and contain a patient's behavior the intervention could potentially produce an adverse reaction especially from those for whom confinement was part of their traumatic experience.

In Custody restraints are part of the arsenal of interventions available to staff when dealing with inmates who might be disruptive and at risk of harming themselves or others. If staff deem this intervention to be necessary, it is important to be cognizant of whether or not the inmate has previously experienced a similar traumatic event and how this action might re-trigger traumatic memories. It is recommended mental and medical staff monitor the inmate regularly to ensure a rapid response were any issues to surface in reaction to possible re-traumatization. It is also important they intervene with the inmate to ensure the experience is processed accurately and re-traumatization minimized.

If the inmate is sent to solitary confinement or segregation and we are aware this intervention might trigger memories of his/her traumatic event we need to acknowledge this by following up with a variety of procedures to include regular monitoring by that person's custody team as well as by mental health and medical services.

The SIX Key principles of TIA are as follows:

A) **Safety-** The organization needs to be committed to ensuring staff and participant physical safety. However, safety refers not only to physical safety but psychological as well. Very importantly, staff's interactions need to promote a sense of safety at both levels, psychological as well as physical.

In Custody, our policies typically address safety of staff and inmates. However, while the objective nature of physical safety can be measured and documented it is less so with psychological safety allowing for this area to be less defined or focused.

This neglect can be attributed to multiple factors:

   a) Psychological safety can be an elusive concept with multiple meanings and expressions. Until there is a solid definition of the concept that would allow others to conduct research it is difficult to monitor to ensure compliance with this directive.
   b) Psychological safety assumes trust and equal power distribution among its members which goes counter to the roles of those in a custody environment where staff have all the authority. It is difficult to trust others who are not equal in power and who are perceived primarily as "jailers," "disciplinarians," and "hostile."
   c) In order to assess psychological safety, we would need to understand how those affected are feeling. However, our society typically has rules for the display of emotions, and/or their acknowledgement. For examples, boys learn at an early age that they should not feel or express "powerless" emotions (sadness, fear). In response to such teachings men learn to interpret the presence and expression of these emotions as a sign of weakness. Men learn early on that "powerless" emotions lead to ridicule

or reprimands. As they were growing up they might have witnessed other young boys being belittled or victimized for expressing their emotions learning at an early age that the expression of emotions is a liability (Safdar, et al., 2009).

d) Custody tends to be predominantly a "male" field at the staff and inmate level. When men are placed in custody they bring with them society's prevailing attitudes pertaining to the presence and expression of emotions with male staff responding accordingly. This interaction perpetuates the rejection of "powerless" emotions.

e) While in custody men are in an environment that is potentially dangerous. The expression and recognition of emotions could be interpreted as a sign of vulnerability in an environment where others would capitalize on such perceived weakness. For the sake of their safety, men have learned to withhold their emotions. This attitude, therefore, makes it difficult to monitor "psychological safety" among male inmates.

f) Female inmates tend to be more expressive and seek more support from others to include staff. This approach to their emotions makes it easier to gage "psychological safety" with female inmates (Safdar, et al, 2009).

Despite cultural expectations, staff can effectively monitor "psychological safety." The following are some suggestions:

1) Publicize the importance of physical and psychological safety through orientation talks with inmates upon arrival.

2) Ensure official interactions include the importance of psychological and physical safety with steps to be implemented if someone does not feel safe.

3) Ensure that when someone does not feel safe they are listened to and that measures implemented safeguard the inmate, staff, and policies.

4) Brainstorm with inmates regarding procedures that might increase feelings of safety.

5) Promote communication courses that discuss feelings, acknowledging their presence, and learning how to effectively communicate them.

6) Promote classes that address victimization, bullying, and consequences of these behaviors in prison.

7) Ensure that inmate's team are responsive and consistent in their approach.
8) One-on-one interviews to assess inmates' psychological safety.
9) Questionnaires inquiring how psychologically safe inmates feel.

In addition, we need to ensure the inmate is feeling safe from recurring symptoms associated with a traumatic incident. We need to inquire if they are experiencing horrifying nightmares, if they are waking up startled, if they are walking in their sleep, experiencing intrusive memories, etc.

SAMHSA (Trauma Informed Care in Behavioral Health Services, 2014, pg. 113) offers five strategies to help in this regard. These strategies are:

Strategy #1: Teach clients how and when to use "grounding" exercises when they feel unsafe or overwhelmed. "Grounding" refers to aiding a person to remain in the "here and now" instead of being swept away by the power of their traumatic memories. This can be achieved by acknowledging what they are experiencing while at the same time helping them remain focused on the present. For example, asking the inmate to state what they are feeling while helping them understand that those memories are in the past, and then asking them to describe their immediate surroundings helps them move into the "here and now" where they are no longer threatened.

Strategy #2: Establish some specific routines in individual, group, or family therapy (e.g., have an opening ritual or routine when starting and ending a group session). A structured setting can provide a sense of safety and familiarity for clients with histories of trauma. Furthermore, when they are in a work environment or group therapy session the structure imparted during that experience helps the inmate learn stability and feel safe.

Strategy #3: Facilitate a discussion on safe and unsafe behaviors. Have clients identify, on paper, behaviors that promote safety and behaviors that feel unsafe for them.

Strategy #4: Ensure staff are prepared for their sessions (or meetings) and they maintain the same format, that the content is predictable, handouts are available, and guidelines are discussed with the inmates.

Strategy #5: Encourage the development of a safety plan. Depending on the type of trauma, per-sonal safety can be an issue; work with the client to develop a plan that will help him or her feel in control and be prepared for the unexpected triggers that might elicit a reaction.

A) **Trustworthiness and Transparency-** A "Trauma Informed Approach" requires for the organization to implement policies that are transparent and promote trust among the participants.

   In Custody, we strive for trustworthiness and transparency. Policies are designed so that each member of the organization understands how the institution operates. This knowledge promotes a sense of stability and safety that is important not only to staff but also to inmates.

   This does not preclude those instances when, in order to protect an individual or the safety of the institution, information is concealed. The most classic example would be that of an individual in the witness security program. To ensure that inmate's safety it is important to safeguard their true identity.

   Institutions can be perceived as being neglectful of this element when their own policies appear to be violated with no reasonable explanation being offered. The same can be said about ignored procedures. When policies are violated, procedures ignored, new rules implemented without any type of formal and reasonable explanation the institution's trustworthiness and transparency can suffer.

   Some suggestions on how to address this issue:
   1) Ensure everyone adheres to policies and regulations.
   2) Be consistent in enforcing policies and regulations.
   3) Communicate in writing all policies and regulations along with reprimands (levels) for not abiding by them.
   4) If new policies are to be implemented put these in writing and hold meetings with those affected before they are executed.

B) **Peer Support-** A " Trauma Informed Approach" stresses the importance of peers helping peers, collaborating in the recovery process, and sharing experiences to aid in their shared healing. ("Peers" refers to those who have being traumatized.)

Ordinarily, institutions offer courses designed to promote psychological well- being. However, in order to meet this requirement inmates need to be able to participate in groups that address trauma and victimization exclusively and primarily. In other words, it cannot be assumed this topic will be covered as part of other therapeutic groups that touch on themes such as "anxiety disorders," "depression, " etc. Instead, institutions need to provide courses that focus entirely on trauma and recovery to meet this key element.

C) **Collaboration and Mutuality–** At first glance, this element might appear to be difficult for institutions to adapt if not entirely impossible because it refers to "leveling" the power differential among staff and participants, or in a prison system, among staff and inmates. For obvious reasons, a strict adherence to this concept cannot be enforced in a custody setting.

However, staff can acknowledge that power differential exists and needs to exist while showing respect to, and ensuring the dignity of, inmates. By treating inmates with respect, which is indeed a core tenet of custody, and eschewing coercive routine interactions, the inmate is validated which in of itself can be a therapeutic experience.

D) **Empowerment: Voice and Choice-** To achieve this element, the institution needs to focus on the inmates' strengths and foster their ability to express themselves. According to SAMHSA, individuals who have been victimized often times have a "diminished voice" (2014, pg 11) and are not supported in their attempts at self-reliance.

This element might be difficult to implement in custody due to the very realistic power differential that exists. However, it is possible to implement in therapeutic groups. Likewise, in those therapeutic groups the inmate can find "his/her" voice and learn to express him/herself appropriately within a correctional environment.

E) **Cultural, Historical, Gender Issues-** Trauma Informed Approach states that it is important for organizations to transcend social mores and cultural stereotypes by incorporating and recognizing the racial, ethnic, and cultural backgrounds of those being served. Corrections staff more often than not receive training on cultural sensitivity. Nevertheless, it is important to ensure that this awareness remains present at all times and this can be accomplished by recognizing, on a regular basis, individuals from different cultures, races, and ethnicity who have made indelible contributions to society. This can be achieved by offering programs that teach about different cultures, bringing guest speakers who address this issue, encouraging exchange of information with custody staff from other countries, etc.

RE-TRAUMATIZATION

As a result of the individual's particular history with trauma it is possible s/he will interpret custody type interventions or procedures in a negative manner if they in any way resemble their previous traumatic experience. This, unfortunately, results in re-traumatization and might make them feel threatened, unsafe and in a dangerous situation even though this might not be the case. They might express feeling out of control and trapped.

In custody, inmates' are monitored almost 100% percentage of the time. The observations staff make can provide valuable information pertaining to inmates' reactions to even the most "mundane" procedures. After all, staff are vigilant of inmates' in classroom settings, at work, in the recreation areas, cells and dorms, etc. It is within these contexts, for example, that staff might observe behaviors that do not seem to correspond to the situation. If an individual responds oddly when going to the dining room it might be worthwhile to inquire since it might be a response to a prior traumatic event.

It is also important to remember that it is difficult to anticipate or predict the types of behaviors inmates might respond to due to the wide range of traumatic situations. All we can do is monitor their reactions and refer accordingly.

Steps that would assist in minimizing re-traumatization include ensuring staff:

1) Learn as much as possible of the inmates they supervise.
2) Learn as much as possible about traumatic events and what signs prompt traumatic reactions.

3) Maintain a good working relationship with inmates without compromising their ability to supervise and discipline.
4) Let inmates know they are available while maintaining strict boundaries.

Interactive Questions-
Form small discussion groups to answer these questions and then role play as if discussing with someone who has not participated in the training. Afterward, meet as a large group. Each team will select a representative who will answer one of these questions in front of the larger group.

1- *Why is the concept of "CONTEXT" important for TIA?*
2- *What are TIA's 4 "Rs?"*
3- *How can our interventions re-traumatize an inmate?*
4- *Develop a list of interventions to aid an inmate who has been placed in solitary confinement feel "psychologically safe."*
5- *Assuming you're the Food Foreman, you're a man, in charge of a female inmate who often cries and you learn she has a history of repeated abuse...how would you approach her?*
6- *You have to place an inmate in restraints and you know she has been victimized in this manner in the past. What reactions can you anticipate and how could you prevent re-traumatization?*

TIA INTERVENTIONS IN CUSTODY

Safety- As stated earlier, the concept of "safety" is paramount to "TIA" and as such it needs to also be a key element for those correctional facilities interested in operating in a manner consistent with a "TIA" philosophy.

"Safety" implies physical as well as psychological safety. In order to ensure inmates feel safe each institution, with its unique characteristics and population, has to develop strategies that will provide inmates, and staff with information pertaining to physical and psychological safety. The institution needs to design interventions geared toward promoting safety, as well as actions for when inmates' report not feeling safe.

Recovery- Recovery needs to become a top priority and the first step toward recovery involves recognition of a problem. However, it is not unusual for some inmates to resist acknowledging the presence of a substance abuse problem or even the possible connection between their substance abuse and their traumatic event. The reasons for this resistance might be multiple. For example, the inmate might feel that once they start addressing the incident he/she might not be able to contain his/her emotions. Some might feel that it is still too recent and too painful to discuss. Sometimes the individual has made it a point to forget the traumatic event so when asked to discuss it this request runs counter to their coping style. In other words, talking about the trauma would be to go against a well-established, ingrained practice.

But, it is important to address trauma because some individuals fail to see a connection between their trauma and their mental health or substance abuse issues. It is not until they have allowed themselves to explore the traumatic event and subsequent substance abuse issues that they might start making the connections that will place them on the path to recovery.

Recovery needs to be addressed by staff who have been trained to approach this subject. If the institution has a mental health department this is where the inmate needs to be referred. The inmates' counselors and case managers might also be in a position to provide these services as long as they have been adequately trained. The rest of the institution should be on board in ensuring that inmates understand that their recovery is of upmost importance to all.

Clear Guidelines and Role Expectations– In a correctional environment all staff, and inmates, have clear goals and role expectations. In fact, staff need to remain focused and not deviate from his/her assigned duties in order to meet departmental goals. Therefore, staff who detect signs of trauma in inmates under their supervision are not tasked with offering therapeutic services. Instead, they need to refer accordingly. Likewise, they need to be aware that if an inmate reacts erratically or strangely such behavior might not exclusively be a result of antisocial tendencies but could very well be due to previous trauma. It is best to refer those inmates to a mental health provider who would be in a better position to address these concerns and indicate if the disruptive behavior is trauma related or not.

Support Control, Choice, and Autonomy- As stated previously, sometimes some individuals rather not confront their traumatic event and this decision needs to be respected. By accepting their decision the counselor is supporting and empowering the individual. This in turn, is affirming that they (the victims) are competent and capable of making decisions and are in control of their lives.

Familiarize Inmates with Trauma Informed Services- It is important to assume inmates have not experienced Trauma Informed Services before and are not familiarized with the concepts or philosophy. By explaining these services to them as part of an intake process and through further training inmates might gradually become predisposed to embrace this philosophy, even if initially they were reticent of doing so. This might allow them to be more candid about the trauma they experienced and lead them to seek help for their symptoms.

Promote Resiliency- Individuals who have experienced trauma have developed a series of coping strategies that might have been useful and life saving at one point in time but are not necessarily adaptive once the traumatic event has ceased to exist. While it is important to note those behaviors are no longer useful and need to be discarded, it is equally important to recognize how at one time they allowed the person to thrive, succeed, and cope. By focusing on the individual's resiliency, one is promoting that person's strengths and resourcefulness. This particular intervention can be implemented by any staff who is familiar with the inmate. In fact, focusing exclusively on problematic areas can undermine the inmate's sense of competency. Focusing on resiliency implies trusting the inmate can succeed and do better in the future.

Promote Hope– It is crucial for those counselors working with traumatized individuals to promote hope. By focusing on the inmate's resiliency and ability to assert themselves in appropriate manners, one is promoting hope for a better future.

Referrals and Screening Tools– Staff need to obtain screening tools that help identify trauma. These screening tools are just that, for screening purposes and not for diagnosing. Individuals who acknowledge or present symptoms of "trauma" need to be referred for further evaluation and treatment.

Intakes offer a unique opportunity to obtain information because it's a procedure all inmates undergo upon arrival at a correctional facility. At this stage the most important goal is to determine if the person has been exposed to a traumatic event and if s/he is experiencing trauma-related symptoms.

It is strongly recommended that a set of screening questions pertaining to a history of abuse and/or other psychiatric conditions be incorporated to this process with the purpose of determining which inmates need to be referred for further evaluation and possibly treatment.

Questions such as "can you share with me the times you have not felt safe?" help to elicit information that could lead to a discussion of a traumatic incident. If the inmate speaks exclusively about their arrest (or some other topic) staff could always add: "have there been any additional instances?" By gently probing in a compassionate manner it is anticipated that individuals with a prior history of trauma will feel comfortable enough to share their experiences.

A second question to incorporate is more direct and it is whether they have ever experienced a traumatic event. This question can be followed up by inquiring if there is an instance in their life they are constantly trying to forget; if they have spotty memories for any particular incident that they felt was "difficult;" if they notice that they have difficulty with their sleeping patterns; if they feel "on edge" often and become quickly agitated, angry, or depressed.

During the intake process, resiliency needs to be emphasized as a means of strengthening the individual psychologically. During intake it is important to inquire how they were able to survive and what strategies they believe helped them cope with the traumatic event. These strategies need to be recognized and if they are maladaptive, recognized for the purpose they once served: to cope with a horrifying situation.

In addition, the following questions need to be incorporated: whether they have sought mental health services; if they have a history of suicide attempts; if they have ever considered or are considering suicide; if they have ever heard voices or seen things others could not; if they have a history of substance abuse; if they have difficulty controlling their outbursts of anger; if they have used psychotropic medications and type; if they have a support system; if they know how to access behavioral health services.

It is important to remember this process is only for screening- a quick review of symptoms to determine if further assessments are required. If the individual decides to open up and speak openly about their traumatic event that is fine but not required at this time. They can do this with their therapist.

TYPES OF TRAUMA

A) **Nature vs Human Caused-** Traumatic events are divided into two categories: natural or human caused. This distinction is important because research has demonstrated people respond differently in the aftermath depending on whether or not the traumatic event was an act of nature or executed with the intention to injure, inflict pain, or kill someone. Traumas understood to have been intentionally harmful are significantly more traumatic to individuals and their communities.

Human caused traumatic events have significantly harsher consequences for the victim(s). Their recovery period tends to be more difficult, they exhibit more problems in their interpersonal relations and have problems regulating their emotions. (Courtois, 2004)

Recovery from natural events, or those that occurred without human intervention (weather patterns, flooding, spontaneous fires, etc.) will depend on the severity of the devastation, amount of time before resources arrive, and length of time feeling vulnerable.

https://www.youtube.com/watch?v=RGa_i_QBO9U
(2:44 minutes)

B) Individual, Group, Community, and Mass Traumas

Individual trauma refers to an incident that affects only one individual. This traumatic event can be single (rape, assault, work related injury) or multiple and protracted (e.g. a life-threatening illness, multiple sexual assaults). However, despite the fact the incident occurred to only one individual, those who know that person, who belong to that person's social circle, who come into contact with that person will also be affected and experience repercussions from the event. Their experiences and reactions need to be acknowledged as much as those of the victims.

Often times, individuals who experience individual trauma feel shame and fail to procure the assistance they require. Unfortunately, they sometimes feel guilty or responsible for the incident. These feelings sometimes lead the individual to not reveal what happened to them and this in turn impedes their ability to obtain the help they require.

Physical injuries are the most prevalent type of individual trauma. Sudden, unexpected injuries (excessive alcohol and alcohol related injuries, gunshot, stabbings, etc.) can have long-lasting health related consequences in addition to extensive psychological repercussions. If the psychological aspects of trauma are not tended to along with the physical ones, the individual, and his/her family, might be exposed to enduring trauma related symptomatology that could have been prevented or ameliorated with early intervention.

https://www.youtube.com/watch?v=VFcKP-1iKns
(15 minutes)

Group Trauma

Group trauma pertains to a group of individuals who are, as a group, exposed to a traumatic event. These are first responders, medical personnel, firefighters, even a gang who has lost team members as a result of deaths.

These individuals tend to resort to each other for support and understanding believing that others from outside the group will be unable to understand them or help them. Sometimes the expression or acknowledgement of emotions is discouraged because they need to complete a task and by the time the task is completed they might be less inclined to seek help. In fact, sometimes the group members might discourage a display or recognition of emotions because it might provoke the other members to struggle with their own emotions.

Mass Trauma

Mass traumas refer to large-scale natural and human caused disasters. Examples would be massive earthquakes, tsunamis, or a nuclear reactor meltdown. Any one of these not only involve the initial trauma, they provoke a series of additional traumas afterwards. For example, after surviving a hurricane, individuals might have to struggle to find shelter, food, water, medicines, other family members, as well as assistance. These other pressures are further sources of trauma for an already traumatized individual.

In mass trauma it is common for the stigma of trauma, and the isolation common to those who have been victimized, to be removed as large number of people are sharing a common tragedy. Ordinarily these individuals obtain significant amounts of support initially but as the public's attention wanes, and helping agencies decrease, the traumatized individual might feel at a loss without the mechanism or resources needed to rebuild his/her life. This, in turn, can lead to re-traumatization.

Interpersonal Trauma – This type of trauma pertains to events that occur ordinarily between two individuals who have some type of relationship. Under this classification we would find Intimate Partner Violence (IPV), which pertains to threats or actual physical, sexual and/or emotional abuse from one individual to another. These behaviors, unfortunately, are rarely isolated (rarely a one time occurrence) and women have been found to be the most common victims of this type of crime.

C) Developmental Traumas

This type of trauma pertains to events or incidents that occur within a particular developmental stage that has a bearing on that individual's subsequent emotional and physical well-being.

Some of these traumas pertain to sexual, physical, or emotional abuse and neglect. Whether these incidents occur once or more than once, they can result in physical, mental and substance abuse disorders that increase the risk of further traumatization inhibiting the individual's ability to meet the necessary challenges and tasks of subsequent developmental stages.

For example, an adolescent who is kidnapped might have difficulty finding employment or establishing an adult like relationship later in life –goals that would be consistent with their next stage of development.

These types of developmental problems arise most likely because the individual was too young to have a sense of identity to revert back to after the traumatic event, or lacked a multitude of life experiences from which to select the best response to the traumatic incident. Furthermore, the young victim might develop distortions about other's and the world that might hinder their ability to adapt successfully to their next stage of development (Courtois, 2004).

D) Political Terror and War

Refugees are individuals who leave their country because they are escaping war, persecution, and terrorist activity. They differ from immigrants because the latter willingly left their home in search of new or better opportunities. Refugees, on the other hand, leave under duress, and their "escape" is marked by fear of death, of torture, of persecution. According to research, "torture" is the event that leaves individuals at most risk of suffering from PTSD (Steel, et al, 2009).

The primary goal of torture is to inflict excruciating pain or suffering to extract information from an unwilling subject or as punishment for belonging to a movement or group. Different methods are employed and are characterized for being demeaning, humiliating, and painful. These methods are employed as the torturer tries to gain total control over the victim to break their will and personality. In order to survive, the victim gives up their sense of self which can result in lasting trauma long after they are no longer being tortured (O'Mara, 2015).

https://www.youtube.com/watch?v=f8HWCh85P9c
(2 minutes)

https://www.youtube.com/watch?v=8cAoxxjw8dI (3 minutes)

E) Combat Trauma

The U.S. military, with its vast financial and human resources, has conducted the most extensive studies on combat trauma. The most salient results reveal, war after war, that individuals who are in combat and are wounded are at higher risk of developing PTSD than others who did not engage in combat or were wounded.

Interestingly, although women's role in combat has continued to increase, men are at higher risk than women of developing Combat PTSD (Trauma Informed Care in Behavioral Health Services, 2014).

Shell Shock Trauma – WWI
https://www.youtube.com/watch?v=S7Jll9_EiyA (1 minute)
https://www.youtube.com/watch?v=faM42KMeB5Q
(50 minutes)

Shell Shock Trauma ("War Neurosis")- WWII
https://www.youtube.com/watch?v=OUumA6VZh8Q
(50 minutes)

F) Historical Trauma

Historical trauma is also referred to as "generational trauma," and it pertains to incidents that are so widespread they affect a whole culture to the point that it influences future generations.

This type of trauma was first identified among survivors of the Holocaust. Research, anecdotes, works of literature helped to explore how generations of descendants of Holocaust survivors continued to be psychologically affected by the trauma that affected their parents and/or grandparents or other close relatives. Work with Native Americans and African Americans also revealed similarities with the descendants of Holocaust survivors. Consequently, it is important to be sensitive as to how historical trauma may have a role in victimizing future generations (Trauma Informed Care in Behavioral Health Services, 2014).

Sotero (2006, p. 94-95) defines this concept as: the "deliberate and systematic infliction of trauma upon a target population by a subjugating, dominant population; (2) trauma is not limited to a single catastrophic event, but continues over an extended period of time; (3) traumatic events reverberate throughout the population, creating a universal experience of trauma; and (4) the magnitude of the trauma experience derails the population from its natural, projected historical course resulting in a legacy of physical, psychological, social and economic disparities that persist across generations."

Interestingly enough, however, research is now suggesting that those who are able to retain some type of continuity with the affected relatives, their community, culture, and spiritual system fare better than those who end up completely disconnected. A study conducted with the survivors of Joseph Stalin's "purge" found that those families who maintained a sense of connection and continuity with the affected grandparents experienced fewer negative effects than those who were emotionally or physically separated from their grandparents (Baker and Gippenreiter, 1998).

Additionally, some "cultural paradigms" appear to protect future generations from trauma. For example, Kidron (2012) found that generations of descendants of Holocaust survivors reported little effect from their grandparents' trauma as long as they felt empowered by keeping those memories alive. In contrast, a completely different strategy but equally effective has been assumed by those whose parents and relatives were affected by the Cambodian Khmer Rouge. In their case instead of keeping that history of persecution alive they have chosen to forget it, in accordance with their Buddhist beliefs, and instead focus on the future. This strategy has helped future generations become resilient and experience less trauma related symptoms than would have been anticipated.

https://www.youtube.com/watch?v=Unm563Eeq-c (2 minutes)

Interactive Questions-

Form small discussion groups to answer these questions and then role play as if discussing with someone who has not participated in the training. Afterward, meet as a large group. Each team will select a representative who will answer one of these questions in front of the larger group.

1- *What is TIA's top priority?*
2- *How do we incorporate Custody's role with TIA's expectations?*
3- *You have a male inmate who was repeatedly raped as a child. He now works for you and is always angry. How would you approach this situation?*
4- *You supervise an inmate who lost his family to Hurricane Matthew. You know he is always getting disciplined for drinking "hooch." How would you approach him?*
5- *Role Play- You have a female inmate from a country where her mother and grandmother were victimized routinely because they did not have legal protection. Her mother and grandmother belonged to a marginalized group. You notice she is withdrawn and resorts to cutting her arms fairly frequently. How would you approach her?*

DISCUSSING TRAUMA

The more we learn about trauma the more we understand that it has many different components and expressions. Let's look at some definitions and distinctions in the realm of "trauma."

Trauma

According to SAMHSA, "**Trauma**" refers to "experiences that cause intense physical and psychological stress reactions. Trauma results from an event, series of events, or set of circumstances that are experienced by an individual as physically or emotionally harmful or threatening and that have lasting adverse effects on the individual's functioning and physical, social, emotional, or spiritual well-being (Substance Abuse and Mental Health Services Administration [SAMHSA], Trauma and Justices Strategic Initiative, 2012, p.2).

According to the DSM-5, trauma is defined as when an individual person is exposed to "actual or threatened death, serious injury, or sexual violence" (APA, 2013, p. 271).

Acute Stress Disorder

According to the Diagnostic and Statistical Manual of Mental Disorders, 5th edition, Acute Stress Disorder results in symptoms lasting from 3 days to 1 month after being exposed to one or more traumatic events (2013, p.281). Typically the response is one of anxiety that includes some form of re-experiencing or reaction to the traumatic event.

When the individual is re-experiencing the incident they may do so by suffering from spontaneous intrusive recollections, dreams, emotional distress, and physical reactions associated with the traumatic event. Some might inadvertently begin to reenact the traumatic incident, and/or avoid any stimuli or situation that reminds him/her of the traumatic event. It is not unusual for the person to experience memory disturbances such as forgetting his/her own address. These individuals can turn their outlook of life and self into a negative one. Sometimes they feel guilty and can become impulsive.

PTSD or Post Traumatic Stress Disorder refers to a psychiatric diagnosis rendered when an individual is exposed to "actual or threatened death, serious injury, or sexual violence" and displays symptoms that extend beyond a month. There are four ways an individual can experience the traumatic event(s): directly, witnessing the event, learning about the event, learning about the event, or through repeated or extreme exposure to aversive details of the traumatic event(s) (APA, 2013, p.271).

Symptoms associated with PTSD involve: a) re-experiencing (dreams, spontaneous memories, flashbacks) b) trying to avoid intrusive thoughts or events that might provoke memories of the traumatic event c) arousal in the form of irritability, difficulty concentrating, sleep pattern disturbance, exaggerated startle response, and hypervigilance d) negative cognitions and mood which refer to an individuals distorted sense of blame and how it affects perception of self.

"**Complex Trauma**" refers to "**Complex PTSD**" or "disorders of extreme stress not otherwise specified" (DESNOS) that account for the organized and complicated array of problems described by those who experience early onset, protracted, and repeated traumatic events usually involving interpersonal victimization. Examples of these complex traumas include torture, childhood abuse, domestic violence, chronic combat exposure, and severe social deprivation.

According to research (Dyer, et al,2009) "These individuals demonstrate at significantly higher levels (a) alterations in regulation of affect and impulses (e.g., excessive risk-taking); (b) alterations in consciousness or attention (e.g., pathological dissociation); (c) alterations in self- perception' (e.g., shame); d) alterations in relations with others' (e.g., distrust, victimizing others); (e) somatization (e.g., unexplained physical complaints); and (f) alterations in systems of meaning (e.g., distorted beliefs). The researchers concluded that most salient symptoms involve self-destructive beliefs and actions to include self-injury, anger, and aggression.

Trauma, PTSD, and Complex Trauma (PTSD) all result in physical, interpersonal, work, and emotional regulation difficulties although at different levels of intensity. For example, trauma is mostly related to physical health problems and some functional impairment (Sledjecski, Speisman, & Dierker, 2008) while those who have been diagnosed with PTSD have significantly lower quality of life and more impairment as evidenced by more depression, arousal, and anxiety. (Doctore, Zoellner. & Feeny, 2011). Individuals who have been diagnosed as suffering from PTSD as well as those presenting symptoms of complex PTSD are known to engage in physical aggression and hostility at an alarming level. (Complex PTSD much more severe than PTSD.)

Needless to say, this type of condition often leaves individual's trying to self-medicate with alcohol and other drugs, licit and illicit.

Factors Affecting Trauma

Not everyone responds the same way to a traumatic event. The wide range of responses is predicated on that person's understanding of the traumatic event and how s/he experienced it. For example, a male correctional officer held hostage might not develop symptoms associated with the traumatic event while another officer, a female, does so after learning she had been fired upon but saved from injury because the gun had jammed. (personal knowledge)

A) Culture
Cultural factors also play a role in the development of symptoms. Some Asian cultures exposed to traumatic events such as tsunamis or earthquakes have found their citizens develop depression and panic disorders while other non-Western cultures developed health-related complications (Trauma Informed Care, 2014).

According to research (Marsella, 2010), "culture" influences the manner an individual provides meaning to the incident which in turn affects the response and its intensity. For example, by providing meaning to symptoms these can be "normalized" or not; by providing meaning to the degree of responsibility (it was "destiny," "fate,") symptoms can be heightened or minimized; by having a general sense based on culture as to how severe or serious the traumatic incident was (e.g. humiliation) and how one is supposed to respond and/or degree of injury associated with the severity of the traumatic event, all of these factors contribute to an individual's response to a traumatic incident.

An individual who is exposed to a traumatic incident such as a natural catastrophe might retain his/her sense of self intact but that same individual might crumble if the traumatic injury involved a targeted attack by another person (e.g. rape, torture, kidnapping) unless their cultural ideas, beliefs, buttress their coping responses.

There is research suggesting that culture plays a strong role in helping even those who have been political prisoners or victims of torture cope effectively with their traumatic incident. According to Johnson and Thompson (2008) research conducted with survivors of political and civil war trauma revealed a wide range of traumatic responses to trauma (from 18% - 90%) and they ascribed this wide range of responses to the manner culture helped them understand what happened to them and to cope in an optimal manner, or not.

B) Gender

Research demonstrates that while men are more likely than women to be exposed to a traumatic incident women are at a higher risk of developing PTSD (at twice the rate) or some of the symptoms associated with PTSD. Most women's trauma is associated with sexual incidents (Kessler, 2000).

Trauma, where an individual fears for her/his life, is associated with more symptoms and more severity of symptoms when the fear of life is associated with human intervention and the possibility of re-occurrence. This finding has been replicated not only with victims of torture but also among the military (Courtois, 2004).

Recently, the media has described a high profile celebrity's mugging. According to the media, five individuals broke into her apartment in the early hours of the morning, tied her hands and ankles, covered her mouth, placed a gun to her head, and departed with millions of dollars worth in jewelry. Since the incident took place she has not engaged in the multiple social events around the world she was known for; she has canceled the shooting of her television program after eight years on the air, a show she once said she hoped would continue on television "forever," and she has not returned to social media outlets because as she has stated "it puts her and her family in harm's way." These types of behavioral changes are indicative of exposure to a highly traumatic incident. These behavioral changes, most likely associated to other inter and intrapersonal changes are consistent with those of individuals who have been traumatized. (http://www.forbes.com/sites/ceciliarodriguez/2016/10/03/kim-kardashians-gunpoint-assault-in-paris-another-blow-to-french-tourism/#1351b328a318)

Risk and Protective Factors

Most individuals exposed to a traumatic event exhibit reactions immediately but more often than not these resolve without long term consequences. The reason for this is because most individuals are pretty hardy and have fairly good coping skills. Let's explore some of these factors that can have a bearing on the degree of trauma someone might experience.

As indicated earlier, not everyone responds to a traumatic incident by developing trauma-related symptoms. In an attempt to explain this phenomena research has determined that individual's have either risk or protective factors that might lead to the emergence of symptoms, or not. Some of the factors that might lead to enhanced symptomatology or their amelioration might be related to cultural factors as noted earlier, but there might also be genetic predispositions, and personal attributes such as better problem-solving skills, stronger social support group, stronger ability to adapt to adversity.

A meta-analytic study of a group of studies (476) revealed seven significant risk factors that might result in PTSD (Ozer, et al, 2003). These seven factors are:

1) A history of trauma
2) Problems with behavioral health prior to trauma
3) A family history of behavioral health disorders
4) A perceived threat to one's life during the traumatic event
5) Perceived social support following the trauma
6) Intensely negative emotional responses immediately following the trauma (e.g. extreme fear, helplessness, horror, shame)
7) Peritraumatic dissociation (i.e., dissociative experiences during or immediately following the trauma)

However, although not listed in the Ozer et al (2003) study another factor to remember is that "gender" is considered a "risk factor" since women are more likely than men to develop posttraumatic stress responses when faced with similar traumatic situations (McDonald, et. al., 2013).

What is "peritraumatic dissociation?" When speaking about this phenomenon we are describing disturbances in awareness, memory, or altered perception during and immediately after a traumatic experience. Individuals report emotional numbing, tunnel vision, difficulty giving the experience understanding, feeling as if they were not in their body and watching everything as if they were in a movie (distortions of self and surrounding), and time either slowing down or moving very quickly. In addition, it is not unusual for them to report amnesia of the traumatic incident.

Research has also explored how the anticipation of "threat" plays into the emergence of peritraumatic dissociation. It appears that a longer wait, a heightened sense of fear, leads to increases in arousal which in turn lead to greater de-realization. (McDonald, et al., 2013). De-realization refers to a feeling of detachment from the world around him/her. We will be discussing de-realization shortly.

Protective factors, as previously stated, refer to those characteristics that make it less probable for an individual to develop trauma-related symptoms. While a wide array of characteristics have been explored and found to be important, the most salient issue that consistently appears to prevent the emergence of, or ameliorate the symptoms of, PTSD symptoms appears to be "social support." Apparently, social support is indispensable when trying to prevent the emergence of PTSD because it influences positively the individual's understanding of the traumatic event as well as their ability to manage the traumatic experience in an optimal way.

In contrast, those individuals who report that the traumatic incident was a turning point in their lives, who have shaped their understanding of themselves and their future within the context of the abuse, who do not have social support, fare worse than those who are optimistic, perceive themselves in control of their lives, and who implement goals separate from the traumatic incident itself (Trauma Informed Care, 2014).

Interactive Questions-
Form small discussion groups to answer these questions and then role play as if discussing with someone who has not participated in the training. Afterward, meet as a large group. Each team will select a representative who will answer one of these questions in front of the larger group.

1- *Explain to someone why there are so many different concepts related to trauma.*
2- *Your inmate is from Latin America and she is telling you that she is traumatized because another inmate touched her buttocks. She describes not being able to sleep, having intrusive thoughts, and crying often. How do you respond?*

3- *This same inmate, how can you engage her resilience coping skills?*
4- *Explain to your co-worker what are de-realization and depersonalization.*
5- *Who are the individual's at higher risk of developing PTSD?*

Responses to Trauma

Individuals who end up exhibiting reactions to a traumatic event might do so in a wide range of ways. Let's explore some of them.

A. Emotional

The manner in which an individual reacts emotionally to a traumatic event will most likely be mediated by their sociocultural context. Initial reactions of fear that surface during the traumatic incident are usually accompanied by shame, anger, and sadness. However, whether or not the individual is able to identify these feelings will depend on his/her cultural view pertaining to emotions. A culture that easily accesses and understands emotions has taught its members to quickly comprehend what they are feeling and those insights can help them mobilize their coping skills. A culture that does not typically recognize emotions might not be in a position to teach its members how to acknowledge troubling feelings and/or how to cope with them. However, members of both groups might be frightened of their feelings if they think they might lead to feeling "out of control." It is not uncommon to find someone simply state they are "numb" because their feelings are so strong and overwhelming it's the only way they can cope with them.

"Numbing" refers to a detachment between emotions and the individual's thoughts, behaviors, and memories. More severe forms of "numbing" can result in dissociative experiences. Someone with "glazed" eyes, sudden flat affect, long periods of silence, speaking in a monotonous voice, exhibiting stereotypical movements, not responding or reacting to the situation at hand, and engaging in "excessive intellectualization, "might be experiencing some form of "dissociation. " It would be wise to immediately refer this person to mental health for a thorough assessment (Trauma Informed Care, 2014).

Dissociation has two components known as de-realization and depersonalization. An individual who feels that the world around him/her does not exist or exists independently of him/her, and feels detached from his/her surroundings is experiencing an episode of "de-realization." On the other hand, when the individual feels detached from him/herself, that person is experiencing "depersonalization." For example, they might indicate that they can see their feet but they do not belong to them. Typically, the individual who is experiencing depersonalization remains socially connected while those experiencing de-realization tend to alienate themselves.

On the other end of the spectrum is "emotional dysregulation" which refers to an individual's inability to modulate his/her emotional responses. These are individuals whose affective reactions are often described as going from "0 to 60" in an instant. Their emotions are so dramatic and intense they are often inappropriate to the context and can result in interpersonal difficulties. These are individuals who due to their inability to restrain their emotional reactions find that each time they "dysregulate" their responses are more and more extreme. Unfortunately these are painful and only become more painful with each episode as they become even more marked, dramatic, and intense. The intensity of these emotions, and their expression, are like a pendulum that swings farther and farther away with each undulation. In prison, emotions such as rage, anger, irritability, sadness might be related to confinement but also to trauma so it would be wise to refer that inmate to mental health for an evaluation.

Research has defined the concept of dysregulation as: (a) an individual's (in)ability to recognize and comprehend his/her emotions b) (un)willingness to admit the presence of negative emotions c) (in)ability to perform and complete goal-directed behaviors and mediate the expression of impulsive behaviors in the context of negative emotions and d) the (in)ability to employ context-appropriate strategies to mediate and express emotions (author's parantheses) (Gratz and Roemer, 2004).

What is interesting is how research has been revealing that individuals exposed to a traumatic incident early in their lives, even when they had a history of adaptive functioning prior to the event, have more difficulty regulating their emotions than those who were exposed to a traumatic incident later on in life. This might be the case because a younger mind is unable to process in an optimal manner the experience (due to their young age they lack the cognitive and personality skills required) and this might in turn lead to maladaptive coping skills and interactions (Ehring & Quack, 2010).

If those individuals who experienced a traumatic incident later in life engage in emotional dysregulation it tends to be short lived and not as dramatic as those who experienced the traumatic event early in their lives. This is the case because they are able to regain their previously held beliefs about themselves and the world, and employ adaptive coping strategies.

It would not be unusual for those individuals trying to cope with dysregulation to seek control over their emotions by engaging in substance abuse. There is evidence showing how NYC residents increased their consumption of cigarettes, alcohol, and marijuana after September 11, 2001. (Resnick, et al., 2004) Likewise, after the Oklahoma City bombing of 1995, residents reported an increase in the rate of alcohol and substance misuse. (North, et al., 1999). Therefore, this is an area that needs to be monitored upon learning someone has been exposed to a traumatic incident- we need to inquire how well they are acknowledging and modulating the expression of their emotions to help them avoid resorting to the use of substances to do it for them.

Suicide: Individuals are prone to committing suicide when they are experiencing intense psychological pain and feel hopeless. These are individuals who believe nothing will change their pain and feel completely despondent. Unfortunately, these beliefs and feelings result in a "tunnel vision" that makes it difficult for them to seek alternatives or explore different options (University of British Columbia, 2013).

Individuals who have experienced traumatic incidents need to be assessed for suicidality. These are individuals who are experiencing extreme psychological one of the major criteria associated with suicidality, and possibly physical pain. If the person is also feeling hopeless about the future they are at increased risk of committing suicide.

Flashbacks- Unfortunately many victims of trauma report what is known as "flashbacks." Flashbacks refer to when the individual" feels and acts as if the traumatic event(s) was (were) recurring. Sometimes there is total absence or recognition of immediate surroundings. These memories are involuntary and very distressful (Brewin, 2015).

The mechanisms that mediate normal, regular, autobiographical memories from those involved in flashbacks seem to be different (Brewin, 2015). For example, it appears that memories are created when an individual focuses his/her attention on objects and scenes in the immediate surrounding that s/he is then able to integrate and store in his/her memory. However, during traumatic events attention becomes like a tunnel vision not allowing the individual to pay attention to their surroundings and the event itself in an integrated manner. Furthermore, it appears that areas that involve sensory and motor movement are activated for traumatic incidents in a manner that regular memories are not (Brewin, 2015).

B. Physical

It is not unusual for individuals who suffer a traumatic experience to initially report physical complaints rather than psychological ones. Ordinarily, the individual is unaware of the connection between their physical ailments and the traumatic incident and it is not until medical tests fail to support the presence of a medical ailment that they are willing to consider a psychological explanation for their symptoms.   Some of the common ailments reported would be pain, difficulty breathing, hyperventilation, sleep disturbance and other symptoms typically associated with hyperarousal.

Hyperarousal occurs when the body prepares itself for a "flight or fight" response and the body's sympathetic nervous system is activated. Hyperarousal is the body's instinctive manner of reacting and protecting itself from a situation that is potentially dangerous. Other symptoms include extreme fatigue, sweating, and/or gastrointestinal distress (Tovian, et. al, 2016).

C. Cognitive

A common disturbance of functioning described by individuals exposed to traumatic incidents involves cognitive changes. Cognition refers to the processes individuals undergo in an attempt to gain knowledge and understanding by employing their senses. Individuals exposed to a traumatic event often describe difficulty concentrating, racing thoughts or intrusive thoughts (a replay of the traumatic incident), distortion of time and space, and memory problems (Yuen, et al, 2012).

When in the presence of an individual who has been exposed to a traumatic event it is important to consider that their sense of self, their understanding of the world, and the way they perceive the future might have been altered in a critical manner. If the cognitions that predominate after the traumatic incident are pessimistic and negative, the individual is at high risk of experiencing distressing symptoms. If, on the other hand, these three areas are addressed and the person is able to generate a series of positive responses, or activate their protective factors, they will be in a strong position to handle their traumatic experience effectively.

Some of the cognitive errors to explore involve: misinterpretation, inappropriate guilt, idealization, trauma-induced hallucinations or delusions, intrusive thoughts and memories. Let's explore each one of these to understand them better.

When we discuss misinterpretation we are referring to assumptions the victims makes regarding how "safe" or "dangerous" a situation might be based on how it resembles the traumatic event. Going to the beach after nearly drowning can lead someone to fear for his/her safety even in shallow water. Going to a parking lot that reminds a rape victim of the parking lot where her assault took place might lead her to believe she is not safe despite police presence in the area.

Inappropriate or excessive guilt occurs when the victim of trauma assumes responsibility for the traumatic experience. This phenomenon is often observed when the victim survives and others failed to do so. It is not uncommon for the victim to feel they should have perished along with the others. Those who exhibit excessive guilt might be feeling responsible for the random act of violence or force of nature that victimized them.

Idealization is when an individual justifies the perpetrators' behavior particularly if this person was a caregiver. This attitude and attachment usually develops spontaneously as part of a survival instinct but is difficult to reconcile afterwards when the whole truth about the relationship emerges. This explains why, in situations like the Stockholm syndrome, some of the victims can show compassion and loyalty toward the hostage-takers (Westcott, 2013).

Trauma induced hallucinations and delusions- These hallucinations and delusions are congruent with the traumatic content. For example, a person might associate the color orange with danger because the person who victimized him/her wore that color often. The connection between the abuse and the color is so obscured that they might be unable to make the necessary connections between both.

Intrusive thoughts and memories refer to thoughts and memories of the traumatic event that trigger strong emotions and behavioral reactions. Sometimes these occur suddenly and unexpectedly without any particular triggers. The individual responds by trying to avoid them or by trying to distract themselves with differing degrees of success.

D. Behavioral

It is not unusual for victims of trauma, particularly when they are young, to reenact the traumatic event. In children this is accomplished as they play and mimic or have their toys relive the traumatic experience. With older children or adults, this reenactment takes a different form and in it's negative expression takes the form of self-harmful behaviors and consumption of substances (Posner et al, 2007). Often, self-harmful behaviors take the form of cutting, picking or burning one's skin, etc. In other instances individuals resort to substance abuse to cope with troubling feelings.

A distinction needs to be made between these self-harm behaviors and suicide attempts. The key distinction is whether or not the individual has a desire to die. If that desire is absent the behavior is not classified as a suicide attempt but is instead understood as "self-harmful behavior." The main goal of self-harmful behavior is to obtain some form of emotional relief by inflicting pain to oneself and experiencing the concomitant resultant behaviors (e.g., feeling relief upon the sight of blood, or burned skin, etc.)

Characteristics of Trauma

Single Trauma- This term refers to trauma that occurs only once. Examples of a single trauma would be the death of a loved one, a car accident, a natural disaster. The fact that an individual is exposed to a single trauma does not minimize the impact of the event on them. If they have had previous experience with traumatic events and are already vulnerable, or the impact of the incident is particularly terrifying, the individual might respond with traumatic stress symptoms and trauma.

In Custody, it could be argued that the process of removing someone from society is tantamount to inflicting "single trauma." Likewise, measures commonly employed in corrections, such as strip searches, forced-cell moves, segregation, restraints, could also be traumatizing.

Correctional institutions committed to the implementation of TIA guidelines need to explore and develop interventions that not only ensure the safety of their facility but also prevent trauma and re-traumatization. Correctional staff need to be mindful of how their interactions and discipline measures might lead to, or exacerbate, trauma.

Repeated Trauma– Traumatic events that occur to an individual more than once are known as "repeated trauma." A particular characteristic of this type of trauma is that it has a "cumulative effect." This means that the person's resiliency or ability to cope slowly wears off. This cumulative effect can result in the person seeking comfort outside him/herself and often finding it in substance abuse, and/or dysfunctional relationships (that initially seem to provide comfort). These individuals' internal resources are so exhausted that often they suffer from medical problems.

Sustained ("Chronic")Trauma- Individuals in chronically traumatic situations have a difficult time gathering their bearings and preparing themselves emotionally before they face a new traumatic incident. This inability to gather emotional strength before being assaulted with a new trauma (literally or figuratively) renders the individual vulnerable and at an increased risk of being unable to employ their resiliency successfully. These individuals are left emotionally and physically fragile, with little internal resources available to initiate positive changes in their lives.

Time- Time to recover from a traumatic event before encountering another is extremely important when trying to gather emotional strength and resiliency. In Custody, we know of individuals who might have been exposed to an extremely violent life style who are then arrested in a traumatizing, violent manner, proceed through a traumatic judiciary process that leads to further traumatizing experiences in prison. We can already anticipate that their reactions once in prison will not be contained or regulated and will most likely be disruptive and antagonistic. These disruptive behaviors need to be addressed as a disciplinary issue but also within the context of trauma.

Losses- As difficult as coping with a traumatic experience can be, the consequences of coping with the losses associated with the traumatic event can be just as devastating. For example, individuals who successfully escape a massive natural disaster report spending months, if not years, trying to recover from the losses sustained. Coping with the loss of a loved ones, losing ones home and source of employment, coping with medical ailments associated with a natural phenomenon (e.g. hurricanes, earthquakes, etc.) can leave an individual disoriented and unfocused for a long time.

Expected or Not?

Learning of anticipated consequences, and preparing for them, gives individuals a sense of control over their lives and the situation. Individuals who ordinarily feel in control of their decisions and outcomes are generally less prone to difficulties coping with traumatic events.

Intentional or Not?

As stated previously, traumatic incidents that were the direct result of someone's intent to provoke pain or injury, typically leaves the victim at high risk of developing trauma related symptoms. The more egregious the traumatic act, the higher the risk of developing symptoms.

While it is a typical reaction for victims of senseless crimes to feel guilty or responsible for the incident, another reaction is for the victim to assign blame and/or to try to find out who was responsible for his/her traumatic incident. This desire to assign blame or find out who/what was responsible can at times become an all- encompassing quest for the traumatized individual. Sometimes this pursuit is accompanied by a belief that unless there is some form of vengeance a "wrong" cannot be "corrected."

These dynamics are, in essence, the individual's attempt to understand, give meaning to, the traumatic incident. These dynamics need to be understood within the context of whether or not they are helping the person heal and recover (Trauma Informed Care, 2014).

Afterward

As stated previously, the traumatic incident is often times not the end of the traumatic incident but the beginning of a series of very emotionally taxing activities. For example, a rape victim has to cope with the subsequent fears associated with the crime; a natural disaster victim has to spend countless hours trying to find food, shelter, sometimes other family members, before even trying to rebuild their own life; a refugee has to contend with adapting to a new country with new mores and new languages, etc. The degree to which an individual's daily routine is disrupted by the traumatic incident oftentimes results in the use of illicit substances, mental disorders, and other behaviors that reveal the individual's weaknesses rather than strengths and, unfortunately, perpetuate emotional and physical weakness.

Timing of Reactions to Trauma

Those who have been exposed to traumatic incidents might react at different times.

Immediate and Delayed Reactions –

Immediate reactions are to be expected in the aftermath of a traumatic event and the sooner the individual reacts, the sooner they can obtain help. For some victims of trauma their reactions might be "delayed." This means it might be weeks, months, or maybe years after the incident before they begin to experience symptoms. Nevertheless, regardless of how soon or late the person exhibits trauma related symptoms, these need to be taken seriously and receive the attention they deserve. Although the symptoms might be "delayed" it does not take away from the fact that they are in response to a traumatic incident and need to be addressed.

There are a number of reactions that can affect the individual who has experienced a traumatic event, as stated previously, and these can range from numbness, nausea, problems concentrating, and restlessness all the way to flashbacks, nightmares, anger and irritability, dysregulation, de-realization, and withdrawal.

Interactive Questions-
Form small discussion groups to answer these questions and then role play as if discussing with someone who has not participated in the training. Afterward, meet as a large group. Each team will select a representative who will answer one of these questions in front of the larger group.

1- *You have a female inmate who will often cut herself because she is "numb." How do you respond?*
2- *Your staff wants to understand what de-realization and depersonalization mean. What would you tell them?*
3- *How does dysregulation "look?" Provide an example.*
4- *Have you ever known anyone who has experienced "flashbacks?" Please elaborate.*
5- *You're asked to speak to your peers on cognitive errors of victims of trauma. What would you say?*
6- *What is the type of trauma that has the most pernicious effects? Can you elaborate?*

Mental Disorders and Trauma

Recent research reveals that exposure to a traumatic incident is the cause of anxiety and depression (Kinderman, et al, 2013).

Anxiety Disorders

According to the DSM5, anxiety disorders share features of "excessive fear and anxiety and related behavioral disturbances. Fear is the emotional response to real and perceived imminent threat, whereas anxiety is anticipation of future threat (APA,2013,p189).

Examples of anxiety disorders in adults would be: specific phobia (marked fear about a specific object or situation); social anxiety disorder (marked fear about one or more social situation in which the individual is exposed to possible scrutiny by others); panic disorder (intense fear that reaches a peak within minutes and during which time the person feels their heart is pounding, they are unable to breath, they are shaky, etc.) and more (APA, 2013, p.189-219). These conditions can be very troubling to the individual as they can interfere in their ability to sustain employment, maintain healthy interpersonal relationships, or enjoy life.

Depressive Disorders

 The common feature of depressive disorders is the presence of sad, empty, or irritable mood accompanied by somatic and cognitive changes that significantly affect the individual's capacity to function (APA, 2013, p 155).

Examples of these disorders in adults are: major depressive disorder (depressed mood most of the day for an extended period of time); persistent depressive disorder (depressive disorder that is present most days for at least 2 years); premenstrual dysphoric disorder (changes in mood associated to a woman's menstrual cycle); substance/medication induced depressive disorder; and depressive disorder due to a medical condition.

Depressive disorders leave the individual with: low levels of energy, little pleasure in life, a negative outlook about themselves and the future, and unfortunately, with the view that they cannot effect any changes in his/her lives. These individuals need therapy in order to stimulate their internal resources that will then energize them.

Cognition and Trauma

Psychological Meaning

As stated previously, people's understanding of the traumatic incident will determine, in many ways, how they will recover from it. If the person views the traumatic incident in a manner that allows them to mobilize their resiliency, then that person will most likely recover sooner and will experience less symptoms than someone who is unable to do so.

Resiliency can be mobilized in several manners. First, by ensuring the person assigns blame where it lies, whether nature or the perpetrator. This is not easy to do, however, and people typically slide into a stance where they blame themselves for what happened to them. This attitude can be countered by monitoring and ensuring the individual remains focused on the present and on how well they've been able to manage an excruciating difficult situation. It is also important to help them set goals, initially easy ones they can achieve, that will help them feel they are still in control of their lives.

Another technique to employ is to teach them to anticipate and expect intrusive memories, physiological reactions (e.g. sleeping and appetite disturbances, etc), aversive reactions, etc. because by doing this these experiences are normalized. Once these reactions are normalized this prevents the individual from thinking and feeling there is something wrong with him/her. This, in turn, allows them to mobilize their "resiliency" which in turn helps them place the traumatic incident within a context of strength rather than weakness.

Disruption of Core Assumptions

According to Frankl (1992) deeply troubling and traumatizing events can lead a person to question and even shatter core beliefs about themselves, the world, and life in general. When these core assumptions are shattered, it is important to monitor how the person grapples with them and we need to ensure they are replaced with beliefs that are life-affirming. If the individual adapts life-affirming beliefs these will assist him/her rebuild their life in a positive manner. If new beliefs center around hope, faith in order, faith in others, optimism about the future, the individual will be able to mobilize his/her resiliency and act from a stance of power rather than weakness.

History of Resiliency

"Resiliency" means how quickly an individual is able to "bounce back" from a negative experience. According to research, some key components to resiliency involve humor, relaxation, and optimistic thinking. In addition, the individual's ability to monitor his/her and other people's feelings and the ability to use that knowledge to make optimal decisions are instrumental resiliency strategies (Tugade and Fredrickson, 2004).

It is important to consider "timing" when addressing the above issues with someone who has been traumatized. If they are depressed, a normal reaction to the trauma, it is unlikely that attempts at humor will be successful. Instead, encouraging the person to engage in relaxation exercises such as meditation or yoga might be a first step toward developing resiliency. Helping the person monitor his/her emotions and those of those around him/her might be another step at building resiliency. An individual who has been traumatized might only employ optimistic thinking and humor after they've had an opportunity to reflect and recover from the traumatic incident.

Interactive Questions-
Form small discussion groups to answer these questions and then role play as if discussing with someone who has not participated in the training. Afterward, meet as a large group. Each team will select a representative who will answer one of these questions in front of the larger group.

1- *An inmate approaches you and tells you he is unable to stop thinking about the stabbing that left him at the edge of death a few years earlier. He tells you he is angry and wanting revenge. He tells you that when he works in the kitchen and sees knives he feels he can't breath and thinks he is going to faint. What do you tell him?*
2- *An inmate tells you she is feeling extremely vulnerable and scared. She tells you that since her rape she feels like garbage that can be disposed. How do you respond?*
3- *How do you elicit a resilient response from these two inmates?*

Sequence of Trauma - REVIEW

As we conclude this portion of our training, let's review some of the salient features of Trauma.

Emotions:

Individuals exposed to a traumatic incident can exhibit a wide range of emotional responses. Each individual will respond in a manner that is unique to them and it is important to not have presuppositions regarding the "right" or "wrong" responses. These emotions can range from crying to seclusion to drinking to abstaining from using substances. Everyone responds in a different manner. Below are some of the more common reactions to a traumatic incident but these are simply examples and not a definite list of all the possible reactions a traumatized individual might exhibit.

Emotional Dysregulation : As stated previously, emotional dysregulation refers to those individuals who are unable to modulate their affective reactions. The concept refers to (a) an individual's ability to recognize and comprehend his/her emotions b) willingness to admit the presence of negative emotions c) ability to perform and complete goal-directed behaviors and mediate the expression of impulsive behaviors in the context of negative emotions and d) the ability to employ context-appropriate strategies to mediate and express emotions. (Gratz and Roemer, 2004)

Individuals who have been exposed to traumatic incidents might be prone to extreme emotional reactions that negatively affect their interpersonal relationships as much as their own emotional stability. Each time the individuals' emotional expression is unrestrained, the more intense the following incident of emotional expression will be. That's why it is so important to help the person learn to modulate their reactions in a positive manner soon after the first episode occurs.

In prison, it is extremely important for both, staff and inmates (albeit for different reasons) to modulate their reactions. Staff, because they need to remain in control of their affective reactions at all times, and inmates because if they do not their reaction can quickly escalate to a physical intervention.

Suicide: Individuals are at high risk of committing suicide when they are under intense emotional pain and feel hopeless. Individuals who have experienced a traumatic incident are typically despondent. If they also become hopeless they are at high risk of committing suicide. It is important to screen for suicide on a regular basis those inmates who have been exposed to a traumatic experience.

Numbing: As indicated earlier, numbing refers to an individual's inability to "feel" or recognize they are experiencing "feelings." "Numbing" occurs when the individual experiences a detachment between his/her emotions and his/her thoughts, behaviors, and memories.

 In Custody it is important to be on the alert for inmates who might exhibit signs of mental illness so they may be referred for proper treatment. "Numbing" would be one of those conditions that alert us of a deeper problem and a referral to mental health services is indicated.

Self-harm and self-destructive behaviors: Occasionally, victims of trauma feel so "numb" they resort to cutting themselves in order to "feel something." This type of behavior is not necessarily "suicidal" because the intent is not in dying and instead, it is in "feeling something." Nevertheless, this behavior is symptomatic of serious mental health issues and the person needs to be referred for an assessment immediately.

Physical Symptoms

Often times the traumatic incident results in long lasting physical problems. For example, someone who was raped might end up receiving surgery or develop a sexually transmitted disease. Someone who was in a natural disaster might have lost a limb. Sometimes the traumatic incident will result in sleep disturbances, neurological disorders, dermatological problems, among others. It is important to recognize that symptomatology related to trauma can be as diverse as the trauma itself.

Cognitive Triad of Traumatic Stress

Individuals who have been the victims of trauma ordinarily express negative views about the world ("the world is a dangerous place and people can't be trusted"), the future (gloomy and dark), and themselves ("I'm damaged," "It was my fault," "I should have handled things differently"). It is important to recognize these thoughts for what they are, reactions to the traumatic event. As these are gently challenged, and the person's resiliency put into action, and with a lot of support, they will be able to implement a more positive approach in their lives.

Triggers and Flashbacks- Research has shown that some colors, music, smells, images might inadvertently remind a trauma victim of the traumatic event. This, in turn, might result in the victim re-living the traumatic event or at least the feelings associated with the traumatic event. Ordinarily, this is a very painful experience for the victim. Flashbacks are very brief but the emotional consequences can last long periods of time.

Dissociation, depersonalization, and de-realization- Dissociation refers to a disconnect between the person's feelings and their thoughts and behaviors. Ordinarily it is understood within the context of depersonalization and derealization. Depersonalization refers to an individual feeling disconnected with him/herself while derealization is a disconnect with their surroundings.

TRAUMA INFORMED APPROACHES IN CORRECTIONS-DO'S AND DON'TS

Now that we have learned the core principles of TIA, understood the different expressions of trauma, learned of the long-term difficulties some of the victims of trauma face, let's direct our attention at how we can implement the guiding principles of TIA in custody.

Principles

The first step an institution needs to take is to be committed to the idea of running a trauma-informed operation. For this to occur, the agency needs to develop an infrastructure that initiates, supports, and monitors the implementation of these initiatives. The agency has to train its staff as well as the population it serves on what "Trauma Informed Care" is and how it will incorporate elements of this modality into its daily operation. A vital component of this transition is for the agency to review policies and procedures that either support TIC or interfere with it as well as to develop plans that monitor the effective delivery of TIC. In order to ensure continuity of compliance, policies need to be implemented requiring training on a regular basis, clinical supervision, feedback, and resource allocation.

Resistance to Change – SocioEcological Issues

Change is never easy and incorporating a new mission into an existing structure is no easy task! This task becomes double difficult when at first glance it appears to run against existing norms.

The largest corrections agency in the US is the Bureau of Prison. Their mission statement indicates:

"It is the mission of the Federal Bureau of Prisons to protect society by confining offenders in the controlled environments of prisons and community-based facilities that are safe, humane, cost-efficient, and appropriately secure, and that provide work and other self-improvement opportunities to assist offenders in becoming law-abiding citizens. " (https://www.bop.gov)

As stated, a correctional officer's primary role is to "confine an offender in a controlled environment..." This premise, however, might appear to run counter to the principles of TIA whose primary mission is to avoid inflicting trauma (as it might happen when officers maintain an offender confined in a controlled environment) or prevent re-traumatization (as can occur when employing the normal arsenal of interventions available in custody).

However, just as correctional officers have become cognizant of the signs and symptoms of a suicidal inmate, as they recognize the symptoms of a mental or physical disorder and promptly respond by referring and obtaining treatment for an inmate, the same can be said about the principles of TIA. With proper training staff can learn about trauma and refer accordingly. Staff can make it a point to learn about the inmates under their supervision and specifically pay attention to those who have been exposed to a traumatic event. Staff can learn to anticipate and/or recognize trauma-related symptoms and refer accordingly. Staff can be cognizant of treatment programs available in their institution as well as in the community. In other words, the correctional officers' role needs to remain in confining an offender in a controlled environment but to that TIA would add "learn about trauma and trauma related symptoms, and how to respond, so you do not traumatize or re-traumatize inmates."

Steps To Facilitate Change

After an agency has committed to TIA principles, it is important to grant authority to a staff member, who belongs to a TIA committee, to initiate and implement changes. This chairperson would be responsible for assessing the implementation of the new initiatives, evaluating the process, and ensuring the agency's policies and procedures reflect the new initiatives.

The committees' role would be to ensure TIA policies are presented to the rest of the staff. Once everyone has been trained, the committee would ensure staff are adhering to the new policies. They would also make themselves available to respond to questions staff might have and be on-site as these changes are incorporated.

Another key step in facilitating change is that of reviewing the agency's policies to identify those that might lead to trauma or re-traumatization. For example, the use of strip searches, restraints and segregation would be areas each agency would need to discuss. Each agency, with its particular requirements, would have to measure these interventions against the backdrop of traumatization and re-traumatization. This dialogue could lead to novel approaches that not only meet the needs of the agency but also remain true to the mission of TIA.

It is important for the agency to conduct a self-examination to determine how effectively it already functions within a trauma-informed context, or how it could improve its operation to meet the principles of TIA. In order to achieve this, it is necessary not only to obtain feedback from the population being served but also from experts in the field of TIA.

As part of the implementation process, it is important to incorporate universal routine screening for trauma. By utilizing a universal screening process staff will be better situated in identifying and referring inmates who appear to have been exposed to a traumatic incident. Early identification allows for prompt treatment that would assist in preventing re-traumatization.

RE-TRAUMATIZATION

Safety

A key tenet of TIA is that of "safety" and it needs to be highlighted when implementing new TIA based policies. Safety speaks to physical as well as emotional safety. Safety issues might require being sensitive to female inmates who are being monitored in the evening by male staff, as well as to male inmates who are asked to strip search after going to the visiting room. Male inmates who were gang raped need to feel secure in the dining hall while female inmates who were victimized in the slave trade and feel powerless need to feel secure while speaking to their custody team.

It is important for staff to obtain input from inmates on how safe they feel in the institution and how could they feel safer. Once staff has obtained this input measures can be implemented that address not only the needs of the agency but also those of the inmate population. Periodic self-assessments can improve these measures that enhance feelings of safety among the inmate population.

The institution needs to provide programs that address trauma and recovery. These programs need to be able to address the whole range of traumas, from individual, to environmental trauma. Programs discussing drug and alcohol abuse need to be incorporated as well. These programs need to be advertised and offered on a regular basis. Community based programs that can complement these programs can be invited to offer services to the inmate population. This collaboration also helps integrate inmates to support services in the community upon their release.

When discussing safety we are also speaking of emotional regulation. Once the individual learns to express his/her emotions " they are able to feel more in control of themselves and will be able to communicate more effectively. Therapeutic modalities addressing emotional dysregulation would include meditation, prayer, exercising, among others.

RESILIENCY

SAMHSA discusses 7 steps to ensure an individual manages and overcomes their trauma-related symptoms (2014). These are as follows:

Focus – by encouraging victims to remain in the "here and now" the individual learns to focus their attention on, and respond to, their immediate surroundings rather than the past. By learning to remain in the "present" the individual begins to substitute "reactions to the present" for the "reactions to the past." This allows the individual to learn how to calm themselves down rather than remain in an agitated emotional state.

Triggers- if the victim is able to recognize those events, smells, situations that might provoke their trauma related symptoms they can anticipate and alter their responses. They can also learn to implement exercises (such as breathing, meditation, etc) that would help them cope with the emotional responses of fear.

Emotion Self-Check- According to SAMHSA, it is important for the victim to recognize two different types of emotions: "alarm" emotions such as fear, panic, hopelessness and "main" emotions such as happiness, hope, love, etc. The first types of emotions provoke extreme discomfort while the second types are positive and provide comfort. By learning to recognize both types of emotions the individual might learn to draw a distinction among them and gravitate in thought and action to those situations (or individuals) that provoke "main" emotions.

Goals – It is important for the victim of trauma to ensure they implement goals in their lives so they don't inadvertently spend most of their time trying to avoid recalling the traumatic event, or employing strategies for coping with a danger that has passed. These new goals need to be a reflection of their dreams and aspirations, of who they are, and what they want for themselves in the future.

Evaluate Thoughts - The individual needs to learn to analyze their thoughts so that when giving in to their fears they can understand their responses for what they are, old responses that were appropriate at one time but not necessarily so in the present. By doing this the individual can start exploring new forms of expressions when they feel scared, lonely, or in panic.

Options- The traumatized individual needs to identify, and learn how to implement, other responses besides "fear" (or "alarm") when a trigger threatens to set off their trauma related symptoms. It might take the individual some time to learn how to substitute such an ingrained response for another but with time they will be able to succeed.

Contribution- Individuals who have been traumatized ordinarily feel shame, hopelessness, and that they are worthless. These attitudes can be confronted by recognizing the individual's positive, personal, attributes and their emotional strengths. Furthermore, the individual needs to be encouraged to contribute to their environment (e.g. participate in peer support groups, donate time to a worthy cause) because as they do so others will react positively which in turn will have a positive effect on their image and boost their self-confidence.

Interactive Questions-
Form small discussion groups to answer these questions and then role play as if discussing with someone who has not participated in the training. Afterward, meet as a large group. Each team will select a representative who will answer one of these questions in front of the larger group.

1- *You are asked to give a presentation on emotional aspects of trauma in prison. How would you explain emotional dysregulation, suicide, numbing, and self-destructive behaviors to staff?*
2- *Your boss asks you to explain how stress affects the body. What would you tell her?*
3- *Your co-worker knows you attended training on Trauma Informed Care and asks you what "triggers and flashbacks" mean? What do you tell him?*
4- *Role play the following scenario: An individual is experiencing an episode of "depersonalization" and you wish to help him/her through it.*
5- *A new inmate tells you that she does not feel "safe" in an open bay dormitory. How do you address this concern? Role Play.*
6- *You have observed an inmate react strongly to the color "orange." You learn that as a child they were kept locked up for long stretches of time in a closet that had been painted "orange." You watch how she starts to hyperventilate, dissociate, and sweat. How do you respond? Role Play.*

For the next part of our workshop, we're going to break into small groups that will have as an assignment the implementation of a Trauma Informed program at their agency.

Groups will be asked to:

1) Name a chairperson and Committee
2) Review existing policies looking for "strengths" (policies consistent with a TIA approach) and "weaknesses (policies that could provoke trauma or perpetuate it).
3) Design new TIA policies to replace "weak" ones.
4) What procedures would you incorporate in inmate's Admission and Orientation that address TIA?
5) Establish a time frame for research, implementation, and evaluation
6) Review existing inmate programs and determine if they are consistent, or not, with TIA principles.
7) Identify community resources

The small groups will then discuss with the larger group their decisions and their rationale for their decisions.

We hope this presentation has been informative as well as provocative. Our greatest wish is that you are able to teach these principles and that you can effect positive change in the life of those sent to you for supervision while under confinement.

REFERENCES

About Us. (2016, October). Retrieved from http://www.samhsa.gov/about-us

Al Jazeera English. [Youtube]. (2012,March 10). Tsunami Survivors struggle to cope. [video file]. Retrieved from: https://www.youtube.com/watch?v=RGa_i_QBO9U

Al Jazeera English. [Youtube]. (2013,August 2). Syria's war children suffer mental illness. [video file]. Retrieved from: https://www.youtube.com/watch?v=f8HWCh85P9c

American Psychiatric Association. (1980). Diagnostic and statistical manual of mental disorders (3rd ed., text rev.). Washington, DC: American Psychiatric Association.

American Psychiatric Association. (2013). *Diagnostic and statistical manual of mental disorders: DSM-5*. Washington, D.C: American Psychiatric Association.

Baker KG, Gippenreiter JB. Stalin's Purge and its impact on Russian families. In: Danieli Y, editor. International Handbook of Multigenerational Legacies of Trauma. New York, NY: Plenum Press; 1998. pp. 403–434.

Brewin, C. R. (2015). Re-experiencing traumatic events in PTSD: new avenues in research on intrusive memories and flashbacks. European Journal of Psychotraumatology, 6, 1-10.

Courtois, C. (2004) Complex Trauma, Complex Reactions: Assessment and Treatment. *Psychotherapy: Theory, Research, Practice, Training*. 41,4,412-425

Dr Allen Brown (2013, November 13). Shell Shock in World War II. Retrieved from Dr Alan Brown: https://www.youtube.com/watch?v=faM42KMeB5Q

Doctore, J.N., Zoellner, L.A., Feeny, N.C. (2011). Predictors of health-related quality of life utilities among persons with posttraumatic stress disorder. Psychiatric *Services*, 62, 272-277.

Dyer, K.F, Dorahy, M. J., Hamilton, G., Corry, M., Shannon, M., MacSherry, A., McRobert, G.,& Elder, R., McElhill, B. (2009). Anger, Aggression, and Self Harm in PTSD and Complex PTSD. *Journal of Clinical Psychology*, 65(10), 1-16.
Retrieved from:
http://s3.amazonaws.com/academia.edu.documents/44672563/Anger_agg ression_and_selfharm_in_PTSD_a20160412-11436-1ceieoq.pdfAWSAccessKeyId=AKIAJ56TQJRTWSMTNPEA&Expires=14768 95704&Signature=9h3uhMi%2BoyZfALb4Juqor4%2FtSr8%3D&response-content-disposition=inline%3B%20filename%3DAnger_aggression_and_self-harm_in_PTSD_a.pdf

Ehring, T. & Quack, D. (2010) Trauma Survivors: The Role of Trauma Type and PTSD Symptom Severity. *Behavior Therapy*, 41, 4, p 587-598.

Emsync12. [Youtube]. (2012,March 22). Bridget Kelly: A Survivor's Story. [video file]. Retrieved from: https://www.youtube.com/watch?v=VFcKP-1iKns

Federal Bureau of Prisons (2016, November). Resources. Retrieved From the Federal Bureau of Prisons website: https://www.bop.gov

Forbes (2016, October 3). Kim Kardashian Robbed At Gunpoint In Paris Exclusive Hotel. Retrieved From: http://www.forbes.com/sites/ ceciliarodriguez/2016/10/03/ kim- kardashians-gunpoint-assault-in-paris-another-blow-to-french-tourism/#1351b328a318.

Frankl, V. (1992). Man's Search for Meaning: An Introduction to Logotherapy. (4th ed.). Boston: Massachussets:Beacon Press.

Gratz, K.L. & Roemer, L. (2004). Multidimensional Assessment of Emotion Regulation and Dysregulation: Development, Factor Structure, and Initial Validation of the Difficulties in Emotion Regulation Scale. Journal of *Psychopathology and Behavioral Assessment.* 26,1, 41-54.

Johnson, H. & Thompson, A. (2008). The development and maintenance of post-traumatic stress disorder (PTSD) in civilian adult survivors of war trauma and torture: A review. *Clinical Psychology Review*, 28, 36-47.

Jordan, J. (2004). Beyond Belief? Police, rape and women's credibility. *Criminal Justice.* 4,1, 29-59.

Kessler, R.C.(2000). Post traumatic stress disorder: The burden to the individual and to society. *Journal of Clinical Psychiatry*, 61, 5, 4-12.

Kidron, Carol A. (2012) Alterity and the Particular Limits of Universalism: Comparing Jewish-Israeli Holocaust and Canadian-Cambodian Genocide Legacies. *Current Anthropology.* 1-10.

Kinderman, P., Schwannauer, M., Pontin, E., Tai, S. (2013). Psychological Processes Mediate the Impact of Familial Risk, Social Circumstances and Life Events on Mental Health. *Pone.*8,10.

Marsella, A. (2010) Ethnocultural Aspects of PTSD: An Overview of Concepts, Issues, and Treatments. *Traumatology*, 12, 4, 17-26.

McDonald, P., Bryant, R.A., Silove, D., Creamer, M. O"Donnell, M., & McFarlane, A.C. (2013). The expectancy of threat and peritraumatic dissociation. *European Journal of Psychotraumatology.* 4,10, 1-13.

National Center for Child Traumatic Stress Network, Child Sexual Abuse Task Force and Research and Practice Core. (2004) *How to Implement trauma-focused cognitive behavioral therapy (TF-CBT)* (Rep. No. Version 2) Durham, NC and Los Angeles: National Center for Child Traumatic Stress.

National Sexual Violence Resource Center (2012) *False Reporting.* Retrieved from the National Sexual Violence Resource Center website:

http://www.nsvrc.org/sites/default/files/Publications_NSVRC_Overview _Fal
se-Reporting.pdf

North, C.S., Nixon, S.J., Shariat, S., Mallonee, S., McMillen C., Spitznagel, E.L., & Smith, E.M. (1999). Psychiatric Disorders Among Survivors of the Oklahoma City Bombing. *Journal of the American Medical Association.* 282,8,755-762.

O'Mara, S. (2015). Why Torture Doesn't Work: The Neuroscience of Interrogation. London, England: Harvard University Press.

On Native Ground. [Youtube]. (2012,February 21) Historical Trauma. [video file]. Retrieved from:
https://www.youtube.com/watch?v=Unm563Eeq-c

Pietrzak, R.H., Goldstein, R.B., Southwick, S.M., and Grant, B.F. (2011). Prevalence and Axis I comorbidity of full and partial posttraumatic stress disorder in the United States: results from Wave 2 of the National Epidemiologic Survey on Alcohol and Related Conditions. *Journal of Anxiety Disorders.* 25, 3. 456-65.

Posner, M., Rothbar, M.K., Sheese, B.E., & Tang, Y. (2007). The anterior cingulate gyrus and the mechanism of self-regulation. *Cognition, Affect, and Behavioral Neuroscience, 7,*4, 391-5.

Resnick, H., Galea, S., Kilpatrick, D., & Vlahov, D. (2004, Winter). Research on Trauma and PTSD in the Aftermath of 9/11. *The National Center of Post-Traumatic Stress Disorder,PTSD Research Quarterly,* 15,1.1-8.

Safdar, S., Friedlmeier, W., Matsumoto, D., Yoo, S.H., Kwantes, C., Kakai, H., Shigemasu, E. (2009). Variations of Emotional Display Rules Within and Across Cultures: A Comparison Between Canada, USA, and Japan. *Canadian Journal of Behavioural Science.* Vol. 41, No. 1, 1–10.

Sledjeski, E.M., Speisman, B., & Dierker, L.C. (2008). Does number of lifetime traumas explain the relationship between PTSD and chronic medical conditions? Answers from the National Comorbidity Survey-Replication (NCS-R). *Journal of Behavioral Medicine, 31,* 341-349.

Sotero, M. (2006). A Conceptual Model of Historical Trauma: Implications for Public Health Practice and Research. *Journal of Health Disparities Research and Practice,* 1,1,93-108.

Steel, Z., Chey, T., Silove, D., Marnane, C., Bryant, R.A., van Ommeren, M. (2009) Association of Torture and Other Potentially Traumatic Events With Mental Health Outcomes Among Populations Exposed to Mass Conflict and Displacement: A Systematic Review and Meta-analysis. *Journal of American Medical Association.* 302, 5, 537 -549

Substance Abuse and Mental Health Services Administration, Trauma and Justice
Strategic Initiative (2012) *SAMHSA's Working definition of trauma and guidance
for trauma-informed approach.* Rockville, MD: Substance Abuse and Mental
Health Services Administration. Retrieved from the Substance Abuse and
Mental Health Services Administration website at:
http://www.samhsa.gov/about-us/who-we-are

Substance Abuse and Mental Health Services Administration. (2014, July). *SAMHSA's
Concept of Trauma and Guidance for a Trauma-Informed Approach. (Publication
Number SMA 14-4884). Rockville, MD.* Substance Abuse and Mental Health
Services Administration.

Substance Abuse and Mental Health Services Administration. (2014, July) *Trauma
Informed Care in Behavioral Health Services. A Treatment Improvement Protocol
(TIP) Series 57. (HHS PublicationNo. SMA 13-4801). Rockville,MD.* Substance
Abuse and Mental Health Services. Retrieved from the SubstanceAbuse and
Mental Health Services Administration website
at:http://store.samhsa.gov/product/SMA14-4884

Substance Abuse and Mental Health Services Administration. (2014, July) *Trauma
Informed Care in Behavioral Health Services. A Review of the Literature.
Rockville,MD.* Substance Abuse and Mental Health Services.Retrieved from
the Substance Abuse and Mental Health Services Administration website at:
http://store.samhsa.gov/product/SMA14-4884

Tedx Talks. [Youtube]. (2015,March 20). The effect of trauma on the brain and how it
affects behaviors: John Rigg. [video file]. Retrieved from:
https://www.youtube.com/watch?v=m9Pg4K1ZKws

Tovian, S., Thorn, B., Coons, H., Labott, S., Burg, M., Surwit, R., & Bruns,D. (2016).
Stress Effects on the Body. *American Psychological Association.* Retrieved
from: http://www.apa.org/helpcenter/stress-body.aspx

Tugade, M. & Fredrickson, B. (2004). Resilient Individuals Use Positive Emotions to
Bounce Back from Negative Emotional Experiences. *Journal of Personality and
Social Psychology.* 86,2, 320 – 333.

University of British Columbia. (2013, June 13). First major study of suicide
motivations to advance prevention. *ScienceDaily.* Retrieved November 25,
2016 from www.sciencedaily.com/releases/2013/06/130613092348.htm

Voice of America. [Youtube]. (2014,May 6) Bringing Healing to Traumatized Victims
of Mass Violence . [video file]. Retrieved from Voice of America:
https://www.youtube.com/watch?v=8cAoxxjw8dI

War Archives. (2011, September 22) Shell Shock Victim, World War I. Retrieved from
War Archives.
https://www.youtube.com/watch?v=S7Jll9_EiyA

Westcott, K. (2013). What is Stockholm Syndrome? Retrieved from: BBC News
Magazine.
http://www.bbc.com/news/magazine-22447726

World Health Organization. (2013, August 6) *WHO releases guidance on mental health care after trauma.* Retrieved from The World Health Organization website: http://www.who.int/mediacentre/news/releases/2013/trauma_mental_health_20130806/en/

Yuen, E., Wei, J., Liu, W., Zhong, P., Li, X., Yan, Z.(2012) Repeated Stress Causes Cognitive Impairment by Suppressing Glutamate Receptor Expression and Function in Prefrontal Cortex . *Neuron.* 73, 962-977.

www.ingramcontent.com/pod-product-compliance
Lightning Source LLC
Chambersburg PA
CBHW070931270326
41927CB00011B/2815